How To Get Rid
Of Allergies Fast

294 Great Tips To Treat And Prevent Allergies

ADAM COLTON

Published by BizMove
www.bizmove.com

294 Great Tips To Treat And Prevent Allergies

An allergy is a reaction by your immune system to something that does not bother most other people. People who have allergies often are sensitive to more than one thing. Substances that often cause reactions are

1. Pollen
2. Dust mites
3. Mold spores
4. Pet dander
5. Food
6. Insect stings
7. Medicines

Normally, your immune system fights germs. It is your body's defense system. In most allergic reactions, however, it is responding to a false alarm. Genes and the environment probably both play a role.

Allergies can cause a variety of symptoms such as a runny nose, sneezing, itching, rashes, swelling, or asthma. Allergies can range from minor to severe. Anaphylaxis is a severe reaction that can be life-threatening. Doctors use skin and blood tests to diagnose allergies. Treatments include medicines, allergy shots, and avoiding the substances that cause the reactions.

While allergic symptoms are already annoying on their own, people who suffer from allergies should not have to worry about the added cost of treating them as well. Learn how to find inexpensive and easy ways to treat your allergy symptoms by reading the helpful tips outlined in this book.

1. To keep allergies under control indoors, you should use an air conditioner so that you do not have to open windows. You should also consider putting a filter in your air conditioner, in order to filter any outdoor impurities that are trying to sneak their way into your home.

2. If you plan to spend time outdoors on windy days, you may find yourself worrying about the effects of pollen on your eyes. One way to protect your eyes is by, donning an oversized pair of sunglasses. Bold wraparound styles are ideal, anything is better than facing airborne allergens head-on.

3. Because mold grows in warm, damp environments, it is very common in organic gardening materials. Compost heaps are a significant source of mold spores and other allergens, which is very frustrating for allergy sufferers who prefer eco-friendly gardening techniques. While composting, always wear a

face mask. This allows you to do your dirty work without having an allergy attack.

4. Keep your pets groomed if you suffer from allergies. Regular brushing not only removes excess hair and dander, but it keeps pets from bringing in pollen from outdoors, too. While it's hard to completely eliminate allergens when you have pets, you can probably your symptoms under control with a bit of extra care.

5. When it comes to getting help from doctors, many people are uncomfortable with the idea of seeking a second opinion or questioning a diagnosis. However, it is true that many doctors spend only a limited time with patients, and may not ask enough questions. Volunteering this information during your appointment may make it easier to find help for your problem. Getting a referral to an allergist, or other specialist.

6. If you find your allergies to be getting unbearable, you may need to look into the possibility of allergy shots. These are available for a wide range of allergies. They can help almost anyone to deal with their allergies more easily. Talk to your doctor to see what options are available to you.

7. If you have allergies, one hidden danger to you may be the damp areas of your home. Places like basements and garages will harbor mold and instigate attacks, so either avoid these areas during the damp season, or see that they are thoroughly cleaned with a simple solution of bleach and water.

8. Keep yourself warm in the winter. Although many people suffer from allergies in warm months, a lot of people still have problems in the winter. A great idea is to bundle-up and cover your nose and mouth so that the air you breathe is warm. That can help you avoid allergy attacks in the winter.

9. One way to keep allergies under control is, to make sure that all of the surfaces in your house are cleaned. This is good to do because you will limit the amount of exposure you will have to dust, and other particles that may cause allergy outbreaks. Limit the amount of chemicals that you use by just cleaning with a damp rag.

10. You can reduce the amount of exposure you have in your home to potential allergens. You should keep your windows, and doors closed to prevent pollen from entering your home. You can take a quick shower after returning from

outdoors to remove pollen from your eyelashes, hair and skin. You should also change clothing and put the clothes that you wore outdoors in closed hamper.

11. If you are someone who is sensitive to getting a lot of allergies, then make sure you always carry some type of cloth or tissue. Do not be that person with a runny nose that does nothing about it. Be prepared at all times.

12. Purchase a portable air purifier, or filter to use throughout your home. Ensure that the device uses at least one HEPA (high-efficiency particulate air) filter to remove allergens from the air you breathe. Place the purifier in your bedroom for a few hours before you go to sleep for an allergy-free night's rest.

13. Use a dust mite cover for your bed and pillows. Many people report dramatic improvement in their allergies when they take this simple step. These cases do not cost much, but they keep dust mites from bothering you as you sleep. Try to avoid plastic cases, because they tend to crinkle and make noise.

14. Wash your hair daily if you suffer from seasonal allergies. Hair collects allergens, and hair styling

products can help your hair trap even more of these things. Allergy problems can be caused by unwashed hair hanging in and around the face. Wash your hair every day to avoid allergen build-up.

15. One way to keep allergies under control is to ensure that you clean your bed sheets on a weekly basis. This is important, because any number of airborne allergies as well as items that you track in can harvest in your bed. You do not want to be exposed to these items, especially with the amount of time spent in bed.

16. There is no need to handle allergies on your own. There is no reason why you should be condemned to a lifetime of sneezing, sniffling and battling your symptoms. If you can't find relief through over-the-counter allergy drugs, then it's time to consult a doctor. Your doctor can prescribe allergy medicine that will relieve you of your symptoms.

17. You may want to reconsider how you dry your clothes. A clothes line is a wonderful place to dry your clothes, but not if you are an allergy sufferer. If you hang our clothes outside, you invite pollen and other irritants from the outdoors on to all your laundry. This can cause a

lot of problems when it increases allergy symptoms.

18. Monitor pollen forecasts and plan accordingly. If you have access to the internet, many of the popular weather forecasting sites have a section dedicated to allergy forecasts including both air quality and pollen counts. On days when the count is going to be high, keep your windows closed and limit your time outdoors.

19. If you suffer from allergies, you need to carefully choose which laundry detergents you use. Certain brands of detergents can trigger allergy symptoms. If you find that all detergents bother your allergies, you could always wash your clothing, and your linens with baking soda. Also, allow your clothing to air dry rather than using a dryer.

20. Wash your hair and take a shower prior to bed. Pollen gathers on your hair and skin and can cause an allergic reaction while you sleep. You will likely sleep much more comfortably if you have a quick shower beforehand.

21. Limit the amount of throw rugs you have around your home. They can gather dust, dirt, pollen, pet dander, and other allergens. If you do

have throw rugs around the home, make sure they are washable. You can do this every week when you are cleaning your home.

22. During certain times of year, people who suffer from allergies have reactions to things in their environment. If you are having symptoms that you think are related to allergens in your environment, consult your physician to try to identify the culprit. Taking over the counter remedies may work to some extent, but you are better off seeing a doctor to advise you on your condition.

23. Allergies can be a confusing condition for many people. People do not understand the difference between real food allergies and standard food intolerances. Allergies are caused by an immune reaction, while the latter is caused by digestion problems. Consult a doctor to find out the cause of your allergies, so you know what causes your condition.

24. When you are taking medications for allergies, it is of critical importance that you consult with your doctor and pharmacist about any foods or other drugs that may not interact properly with your medication. The side effects and reactions between drugs can be extreme, so you need to

know before you take them if there are any risks associated with consuming other drugs or foods.

25. If you experience your allergy symptoms like clockwork, watch that clock. Avoid going out between 5 and 10 o'clock in the morning. This is when pollen is most prevalent. If you have to go out, do not do too much and make your trip quick.

26. Make sure your car is closed and clean to fight allergies. Using the air-conditioner and having all windows closed will prevent pollen from coming inside the car. Regular vacuuming will keep your upholstery and interior free from allergens. This can lessen your allergy problems.

27. If your child is allergic to insect bites and stings, it makes it difficult to participate in outdoor sports and activities. Ask a pediatrician about immunotherapy, an in-office treatment, in which insect venom is introduced to your child's system in increasing amounts. This desensitizes the immune system to stings and gives your child the freedom to join in the outdoor fun.

28. If you are planning a trip, and someone in your party has a severe food allergy. Visit a doctor before departing. Request a prescription for an

extra epinephrine pen to keep with you at all times. To avoid mix-ups, or delays at airport security checkpoints. Keep a copy of the prescription, and directions with the package.

29. Consider taking an over the counter medicine to battle allergy problems. Medicine may clear up any allergy problems you have. Before choosing which medicine is right for you, consult your doctor to make sure it won't affect any medication you are currently taking. Your doctor may also recommend an allergy medicine to you.

30. The use of over-the-counter medication can be effective in treating and controlling allergy symptoms when used correctly. Be sure to take your antihistamine medication before leaving the house in order to allow it to start to work. If you will be driving or doing any activity that requires your attention, be sure to use a non-sedative antihistamine to avoid drowsiness.

31. Shower and change your clothes before going to bed every night. Be sure to thoroughly shampoo your hair. This will eliminate the buildup of allergens you acquire through the day. This also helps from spreading allergens, like dust and pollen, to your bed and making allergy symptoms worse overnight.

32. Try your best to stay away from foods like dairy that can leave you congested. Although you may enjoy yourself very briefly with some rich dairy foods like ice cream. You can pay for it later when with a bad allergic reaction that can leave you congested for days.

33. When you are traveling by car, try your best to keep the windows closed at all times during allergy season. On nice days, many people roll down their car windows to enjoy the weather, but you should avoid doing that and turn on the air conditioner if you need to feel a breeze.

34. Get rid of carpets. Many people who suffer with allergies feel much better after simply ripping up all the carpets in their home and replacing the flooring. If you cannot do this, try to treat your carpets with solutions that can kill dust mites, such as those that contain tannic acid.

35. If you participate in outdoor activities like camping, jogging or team sports, you may need to wash your workout clothes or uniform more frequently than usual-- after every time you wear it, if possible. Some people who are especially sensitive may even become irritated by grass stains, sweat or dirt on their clothing.

36. Allergies can be a confusing condition for many people. People do not understand the difference between real food allergies and standard food intolerances. Allergies are caused by an immune reaction, while the latter is caused by digestion problems. Consult a doctor to find out the cause of your allergies, so you know what causes your condition.

37. Watch your local weather forecast to see if pollen is high for that day. If it is, it's best that you minimize your time spent outdoors. If you do want to go outdoors, make sure it's not between the hours of 5 and 10 A.M. This is the time when pollen is high.

38. If allergies are causing your nose to drip constantly, you might experience chafing, redness and soreness around your nostrils. Using paper tissues to stop drips can make this condition even worse. Instead, discretely dab at your nose with a cotton cloth or handkerchief or apply Vaseline to your nostrils to protect your skin.

39. If you have allergies and are facing yard work, protect yourself with a mask! Any inexpensive painter's mask will help to keep pollen from the

grass and flowers from bothering you. Wear one whenever you have to kick up leaves, mow the lawn or trim hedges, and you should reduce the symptoms you experience.

40. Athletic types who struggle with allergies, often find themselves dreading their daily jog around the neighborhood when pollen counts are high. While some level of pollen will always be in the air at any given time, there is still hope. Pollen content is often at its highest between 5 a.m. and 10 a.m. Choose another period outside of this window, and you should have less trouble.

41. Vacuum your home often. Most homes have at least a few rooms that are carpeted, but carpet is a magnet for allergens and other irritants. An ordinary vaccum is not enough to catch the tiny particles that trigger allergy symptoms. In order for your vacuum to be effective, look for bags or filters that feature a HEPA technology.

42. To keep allergies at bay, try adding a bit of horseradish, or hot mustard to your foods. These act as a natural decongestant. They offer a good alternative to allergy medications, that may cause drowsiness, and morning fatigue. Of course, this is not a good idea for children, as spicy substances can cause them a lot of misery!

43. Make sure the bathrooms in your house remain clean. Bathrooms are a breeding ground for mold, and should be cleaned at least once a week. Use a bleach and water mixture as a cleaning solution to eliminate mold. This cleaning technique will also prevent mold from making allergies worse by growing slowly over time.

44. Try using synthetic pillows over natural or feather pillows. Most dust mites prefer the natural material, so your synthetic pillow should be relatively safe. Even though you must still wash them to rid all the allergens and dust, it is much better for your sleep.

45. Clean your home from top to bottom at least once per year, preferably in the spring. A deep cleaning can eliminate dust, dander, mold and other allergens. If this type of cleaning is too daunting, hire a service to complete the job for you. You can maintain the results yourself or schedule regular visits from the cleaning service, after the initial deep-clean.

46. For allergy sufferers who are especially sensitive to common allergens, it is important to reduce or entirely avoid using the hands to touch their

faces. Surface allergens are easily transferred from the fingers to delicate areas like the mouth, eyes and nasal area. Touching the face with dirty hands may also lead to acne.

47. While an allergy test can be useful in helping you to identifying the culprit of your allergy symptoms, there are certain times in which taking this test is ill-advised. For example, you should never agree to an allergy test when you are experiencing severe asthma symptoms. It is also best to avoid testing while in recovery from surgery, or illness. During these periods, your body may not respond to the tests, as it would in good health.

48. If you are allergic to pollen, always wash your hair before you go to bed. When you are out during the day, pollen can accumulate in your hair. When you go to bed, the pollen will rub off onto your pillow, and will probably end up getting in your nose, eye, and month. This will cause your allergies to flare up.

49. If you experience post-nasal drip as a result of allergies, you may feel as if there is a large amount of mucus in the back of your throat. This uncomfortable feeling is actually the result of a swollen or irritated uvula, and you may end

up with a sore throat if you constantly try to dislodge non-existent mucus. Drink a glass of ice water to reduce that swelling and provide quick relief.

50. If you have a dog or cat that goes outside, make sure to wash him or her as often as possible. Outdoor animals tend to bring in all kinds of things from outside, and pollen is just one of the things they carry. Make sure to clean your pet; if possible, have someone else clean your pet to avoid an allergy attack.

51. If you are one of the millions who suffer from allergies, you probably should change your air filters in your air conditioner every month. The manufacturers usually will say to change every three months, but if you have problem allergies, you should do it more often to ensure all allergens are trapped before being dispersed through your home.

52. Before cementing your plans to spend time in the great outdoors, check the forecast for your location. If the forecast includes high winds, it may be best to reschedule. Windy weather is notorious for stirring up spores and pollen, which could make it difficult to breathe easily while camping, hiking or getting back to nature.

53. Exercise at the right time of day. If you like to exercise outdoors, yet you are an allergy sufferer, there are things that can be done so you can still enjoy the experience. It's better to exercise outdoors in the early morning or later in the evening as the pollen levels aren't as high at these times and less likely to cause issues with your allergies.

54. Your body could be causing an allergic reaction. It's true! You are a magnet for dust and pollen, and pick it up constantly when outdoors. By day's end, you are just coated! If you go to bed without a shower, you will be sleeping with allergens, and you will no doubt, wake up with symptoms. Before going to sleep, you should shower or change your clothes.

55. A good way to reduce your exposure to allergens is to close your windows and doors in the morning and night. Many of the common allergens are at their peak during these times of the day. Most outdoor allergens are pollen. Natural sources like pollen are at their highest levels at these times of the day.

56. If you are going outdoors when allergy season is in full force, wear sunglasses. Sunglasses prevent

pollen, and other allergy triggers from getting in your eyes. About one hour before heading outdoors, put eye drops in your eyes. This will prevent your eyes from getting red when you are outdoors.

57. If you or someone in your family suffers from allergies, prohibit smoking in your car and your home. Smoke is a major allergy trigger for many, and permeates porous surfaces, making it difficult to entirely remove. Ask smokers to step outside before lighting up, and never allow them to smoke inside your vehicle.

58. Slow down. When you find yourself dealing with pet allergies, you may initially be distraught and think you have to give up a beloved pet. The truth is there are many ways to deal with this type of problem without losing your loved one. Talk to a medical professional to see what options you have.

59. Make a saltwater nasal spray at home if you suffer from allergies. This can greatly help any nasal congestion you have. To do this, simply mix a half a teaspoon of salt with 8 ounces of water into a squirt bottle. Then, just use the spray in your nose like you would have with any other nasal spray.

60. Remove all pet hair from upholstery by vacuuming at least once a week. There are some vacuums available with a pet hair attachment that is better at picking up pet hair. Don't allow your pets on your furniture to avoid any build-up of dander or hair in the future.

61. One good way to reduce allergic reactions is to dust your home each week. Some ignore this just until they can see the build-up, but doing it weekly can help reduce your symptoms since it reduces the allergens in your home.

62. Find an allergen forecast and use it to plan your day. The Weather Channel and some other major outlets provide information about pollen activity and other information about allergens. These forecasts can not only let you know which days are likely to be worst for your symptoms, but they can pinpoint the worst times of day to be outside.

63. Skip intense workouts during allergy season. When you are in an intense workout session, you are likely to breathe more deeply, and more quickly. That means you are probably going to inhale much more pollen than usual. Which

means you have a greater chance of experiencing allergy symptoms.

64. Get rid of carpets. Many people who suffer with allergies feel much better after simply ripping up all the carpets in their home and replacing the flooring. If you cannot do this, try to treat your carpets with solutions that can kill dust mites, such as those that contain tannic acid.

65. For people who suffer from seasonal allergies, the best way to reduce your symptoms is to leave the outdoors outside. When you are in your car, drive with the windows up. At home, close windows and use the air conditioner. If you do go outdoors, then you should change your clothes when you come home because it will collect allergens.

66. When your allergies flare, irrigate your sinuses and nasal passages for quick relief from your symptoms. Use a neti pot or other nasal irrigation product along with sterile, filtered, boiled and cooled or distilled water. This practice flushes out irritants and excess mucus, allowing you to breathe more easily.

67. Keep pollen at bay! Pollen can get into your hair. and on your skin without you knowing it.

Try to have a shower, or bath every night. To reduce pollen getting into your home, keep the windows and doors closed whenever possible. Change your air filters regularly during the spring.

68. Reduce your stress level. Stress can be a very significant contributor to allergies, even prolonging the length of attacks far beyond normal. If you suffer from allergies, try to minimize the level of stress you experience or find ways to effectively channel it out of your day. Lowering stress will have a positive outcome on your nagging allergies.

69. Shower before bed, taking special care to wash your hair thoroughly. Pollen, dust, and other allergens can get trapped on your skin and in your hair as you go through your day. If you normally shower in the morning, consider switching to an evening schedule. This will give you the chance to remove these irritants before bed, allowing you to have a restful night's sleep.

70. If you suffer from allergies, you need to carefully choose which laundry detergents you use. Certain brands of detergents can trigger allergy symptoms. If you find that all detergents bother your allergies, you could always wash your

clothing, and your linens with baking soda. Also, allow your clothing to air dry rather than using a dryer.

71. Nice weather often leads to open windows to let air circulate and lower air conditioning bills. This, however, can cause a flare-up of allergy symptoms. To help effectively reduce allergens present in your home, consider installing a HEPA filter in your air conditioning unit. If you have allergies, this will help you to breathe easier.

72. If you have allergies, do not leave the windows open, no matter where you are this. Whether at home, or in the car, keep the windows shut, and put the air conditioner on. Leaving the windows open allows allergy triggers to come in. Which of course, will bother your allergies.

73. If you participate in outdoor activities like camping, jogging or team sports, you may need to wash your workout clothes or uniform more frequently than usual-- after every time you wear it, if possible. Some people who are especially sensitive may even become irritated by grass stains, sweat or dirt on their clothing.

74. Many people experience dull, throbbing headaches as a symptom of their allergies but

overlook the actual cause. Painkillers may offer some relief from the pain but do not address the underlying problem. Even though antihistamines are not considered pain relievers, taking one can treat the allergic reaction itself and therefore, eliminates the headache.

75. If you feel as though you are having issues with dust and dust mites in your mattress, there are mattress sealers available to you. You can put your whole mattress in the plastic. With your sheets, you should never notice the difference of the plastic sheet being there at all.

76. If you plan to spend time outdoors on windy days, you may find yourself worrying about the effects of pollen on your eyes. One way to protect your eyes is by, donning an oversized pair of sunglasses. Bold wraparound styles are ideal, anything is better than facing airborne allergens head-on.

77. Do not use wet methods of cleaning your carpeting or rugs. This can actually increase the number of dust mites it harbors, and it increases the likelihood of mildew growth. Stick to dry cleaning methods, instead, if at all possible. The best way to reduce allergens is to ditch the carpeting altogether.

78. If you use medication to treat allergies, be sure you are using them the right way. A lot of the medication require you to use it for a while before it becomes effective. You will not be able to simply take one dose at the first sign of a sneeze. Speak with your physician about how to use it properly.

79. Sometimes, new clothing can contain chemicals or other allergy-causing substances that can cause a rash or hives upon contact with your skin. When you buy new clothing, be sure to wash each item before you wear it. This is particularly true of man-made materials such as nylon and rayon.

80. When ever you are cleaning your house, use a dust mask. This will help keep away the dust, pollen, and dust mites that are scattered in the air, as you clean out of your system. Most supermarkets have these in the cleaning supplies aisle. If they don't, home improvement stores sell them in bulk.

81. When it comes to getting help from doctors, many people are uncomfortable with the idea of seeking a second opinion or questioning a diagnosis. However, it is true that many doctors

spend only a limited time with patients, and may not ask enough questions. Volunteering this information during your appointment may make it easier to find help for your problem. Getting a referral to an allergist, or other specialist.

82. Relieve symptoms from allergies by taking more vitamin C. Vitamin C is an antihistamine that works be strengthening the immune system. The normal recommended intake for allergy protection is 1000mg daily. Furthermore, foods that are high in Omega-3 are also helpful in treating allergy symptoms.

83. If you suffer from allergies you should vacuum as often as you can. This reduces the amount of allergens that will be floating around your home. For best results, you should also consider certain aspects of the vacuum cleaner itself. Older vacuums are not made to contain microscopic allergens, and could re-spread them into the air. Newer model vacuums come equipped with HEPA filters that can trap over 99% of allergens and small particles to stop them from circulating in the air.

84. If you are one of the millions who suffer from allergies, you probably should change your air filters in your air conditioner every month. The

manufacturers usually will say to change every three months, but if you have problem allergies, you should do it more often to ensure all allergens are trapped before being dispersed through your home.

85. Before cementing your plans to spend time in the great outdoors, check the forecast for your location. If the forecast includes high winds, it may be best to reschedule. Windy weather is notorious for stirring up spores and pollen, which could make it difficult to breathe easily while camping, hiking or getting back to nature.

86. If you suffer from allergies, you need to carefully choose which laundry detergents you use. Certain brands of detergents can trigger allergy symptoms. If you find that all detergents bother your allergies, you could always wash your clothing, and your linens with baking soda. Also, allow your clothing to air dry rather than using a dryer.

87. Shower and wash hair before going to sleep. Your hair and skin can accumulate pollen, causing you to experience an allergic reaction during sleep. A quick clean-up can prevent a nightly episode.

88. Have separate shoes for indoor and outdoor use. If you do a lot of work in your garden or simply enjoy being outdoors, have a pair of shoes set aside specifically for these activities. When it is time to come inside, your shoes, along with the pollen and dust they carry, can be left at the door - minimizing the allergens that make it into your home.

89. If you suffer from allergies, choose a vacuum cleaner with disposable bags. While these vacuums are less ideal environmentally, they tend to be better for allergy sufferers because they trap dust, dander, pollen and more inside, rather than exposing you to the irritants when you empty a canister into the trash.

90. People can be affected by allergies at any age. Many Baby Boomers grew up without access to allergy tests, and other medical resources. They have lived with allergic symptoms for decades. Allergic reactions often manifest differently in seniors than in young people. For example, older adults may experience itching, and mild swelling, but not localized redness. As a result, many assume that the cause of discomfort is something other than allergies. An allergy test can help seniors to identify allergens, and live their golden years to the fullest.

91. If you plan to spend time outdoors on windy days, you may find yourself worrying about the effects of pollen on your eyes. One way to protect your eyes is by, donning an oversized pair of sunglasses. Bold wraparound styles are ideal, anything is better than facing airborne allergens head-on.

92. If you are extremely sensitive to weed pollens, there is a good chance that you may also be sensitive to certain foods. Consuming melons, bananas and chamomile may cross-react with weed pollens, resulting in a tingling, burning or scratchy feeling in the mouth and throat. Approach these foods with caution.

93. People who suffer from food allergies are generally the ones who need to be the most careful. While other types of allergies can be annoying, food allergies tend to be the most fatal. This is especially true of people who suffer from allergies to shellfish or nuts, such as shrimp or hazelnut.

94. Bathrooms are a common source of mold, which can trigger itching and irritation in allergy sufferers. Running an overhead exhaust fan while taking a hot bath or shower reduces moisture in

the air and helps to prevent the growth of mold. Wash bath mats and hand towels frequently with hot water.

95. Make sure you pick out an antiperspirant carefully. Many common ingredients are very harsh chemicals which can aggravate skin, and if you are prone to allergies, these may be even harder on you. Using products that contain these ingredients may wreak havoc on your skin.

96. Up to 30 percent of people who suffer from seasonal allergies may also experience cross-sensitivity after ingesting certain foods. This leads to a tingling, burning or itchy sensation in the throat and may be a result of a reaction between these foods and pollen. If you are allergic to grass pollens, be wary of melons, oranges and tomatoes.

97. Your child may need to have allergy medication at the ready at school. A note from a pediatrician explaining the allergies your child has can be useful. The school should always have extra doses of the medication on hand just in case your child suffers a reaction while in class. You should inform your child's teacher or school nurse of allergy triggers and place a note in his backpack too.

98. If you have tried everything possible to help your allergies and it is still not working, you might want to talk to your doctor about allergy shots. Although there is no cure for allergies, allergy shots have made a huge difference in the lives of many allergy sufferers out there. See if there are shots available for your type of allergies.

99. If you have allergies and have been outdoors, remember to remove the dirty clothes from your bedroom because it most likely picked up some airborne pests when you were outside. Put the clothes in a hamper in a different room, so it is not close to aggravate your symptoms.

100.   There have been studies that have shown that people who suffer from allergies have found relief by incorporating honey in their diet. Although not scientifically proven, it is worth trying. So next time you are at the farmer's market, pick up some local honey and see if it helps reduce your symptoms.

101.   If you are one of the millions who suffer from allergies, you probably should change your air filters in your air conditioner every month. The manufacturers usually will say to change

every three months, but if you have problem allergies, you should do it more often to ensure all allergens are trapped before being dispersed through your home.

102.   If you own pets, bathe them frequently when allergy season arrives. This is especially true for dog owners. Not only, are pets' hair and dander irritants on their own, animal fur is a magnet for pollen floating in the air, allowing these particles to hitch a ride on your pet and invade your home.

103.   Use high-quality, anti-allergen filters in your home heating and cooling system. These filters, which are usually pleated to maximize surface area, remove even the smallest particles of pollen, dander, and other irritants from the air. Because these filters clog more easily than standard filters, you must remember to change them more frequently.

104.   If you are troubled by different allergies in your home, try putting a dehumidifier or two in the common areas of your living space. Reducing the humidity by at least half can really cut down on potential mold growth, and mold is known to be a big contributor to allergies.

105.   Dust mites are everywhere. These microscopic creatures dwell within pillows and mattresses and make their meals on skin flakes that shed and accumulate. Talk about a nightmare! In order to manage this problem, use zippered pillow cases and mattress covers. Then, wash your bedding weekly in hot water, because hot water can kill dust mites.

106.   Do you know that your body can actually be the cause of your allergic reaction? It's really true. As your go through your day, your clothing, hair and body might pick up outdoor dust and pollen. At night, as you retire into bed, your airways can be affected by these items. Shower or put on clean clothing before you lay your head down to rest.

107.   Stay away from small flowers that do not have a lot of color. These flowers are the ones that tend to bother allergies. Larger, brighter flowers, such as the ones that bees and hummingbirds are attracted to, tend to be non-allergenic, so you should be okay around these kinds of flowers.

108.   Pinpoint your allergy triggers in order to prevent your symptoms. Your doctor or allergist can perform blood or skin tests to determine

which substances cause an allergic reaction. This step helps you minimize your exposure to the substances that cause the most discomfort for you. You may also be able to narrow down your treatments to target specific allergens.

109.   If you are allergic to pet dander, designate at least one area in the house as a "pet-free" zone. Your bedroom is the most obvious choice. Keeping this area clean, and free from intrusions by your furry friends can significantly alleviate your allergy symptoms. The alternative, of course, is to designate a single area in which your pet can stay.

110.   A good way to reduce your exposure to allergens is to close your windows and doors in the morning and night. Many of the common allergens are at their peak during these times of the day. Most outdoor allergens are pollen. Natural sources like pollen are at their highest levels at these times of the day.

111.   To reduce the volume allergens in your home, consider changing up your current window coverings. Horizontal blinds are major allergen offenders and are known to collect allergens on the surface of the blinds. Instead, opt for window dressings made from synthetic

materials like acrylic or nylon. Washable roller shades are another good option.

112.   Kitchens are breeding grounds for mold, which can torment would-be chefs who have mold allergies. To discourage the growth and spread of this unwanted intruder, always use an exhaust fan while preparing food on the stove or in the oven. This draws excess moisture from the air, which makes it difficult for mold to grow.

113.   It is important that you watch what you eat and drinks, if you suffer from ragweed allergies. Believe it or not, certain foods and drinks can trigger your ragweed allergy symptoms. Some of the foods you need to avoid include cucumbers, bananas, sunflower seeds, melons, zucchini, and chamomile tea.

114.   For allergy sufferers who are especially sensitive to common allergens, it is important to reduce or entirely avoid using the hands to touch their faces. Surface allergens are easily transferred from the fingers to delicate areas like the mouth, eyes and nasal area. Touching the face with dirty hands may also lead to acne.

115.   If you have a dog or cat that goes outside, make sure to wash him or her as often as

possible. Outdoor animals tend to bring in all kinds of things from outside, and pollen is just one of the things they carry. Make sure to clean your pet; if possible, have someone else clean your pet to avoid an allergy attack.

116.   If your child suffers from allergies, do not allow them to sleep with a non-washable stuffed animal. Of course, they provide your child with a sense of comfort, but they also tend to quickly develop dust mites. Instead, allow your child to sleep with a stuffed animal that is able to be washed.

117.   Talk to your doctor and see if they have any recommendations about what could be causing you to have an allergic reaction. They might help you realize that you have been exposing yourself to a new environment that is causing your body to react in a certain way giving you allergies.

118.   If you are one of the millions who suffer from allergies, you probably should change your air filters in your air conditioner every month. The manufacturers usually will say to change every three months, but if you have problem allergies, you should do it more often to ensure all allergens are trapped before being dispersed through your home.

119.   When traveling in a car, use the air conditioning, and keep the windows closed. This will help seal the allergens out of your car if you need to travel during allergy season. Make sure you set your air conditioner on its recirculate setting, so that you are not bringing in outside air. Aim the vents so they do not blow into your face.

120.   Make an appointment with an allergist, he can tell you exactly what you are allergic to, and then you will be able to stay away from the things that are bothering you. Normally, they do these tests with a series of skin tests to see if you have a reaction.

121.   If you have allergies, do not leave the windows open, no matter where you are this. Whether at home, or in the car, keep the windows shut, and put the air conditioner on. Leaving the windows open allows allergy triggers to come in. Which of course, will bother your allergies.

122.   When you are taking medications for allergies, it is of critical importance that you consult with your doctor and pharmacist about any foods or other drugs that may not interact

properly with your medication. The side effects and reactions between drugs can be extreme, so you need to know before you take them if there are any risks associated with consuming other drugs or foods.

123.　If you continue to have allergy symptoms, keep track of the time. Between 5 a.m. and 10 a.m., pollen levels are at their highest; it is best to stay indoors during this period. When leaving your house cannot be avoided, you should spend as little time as possible outdoors; it also helps to keep activity to a minimum.

124.　Avoid using throw rugs in your home. These can collect dust and mold and can make allergies worse. If you must have rugs in your home, choose ones that can be washed. You should wash them at least once every few weeks to minimize the build up of dust and mold.

125.　Going for a run around the neighborhood may make you feel wonderful and alive, but pollen and spores in the air can quickly spoil the experience. This is especially true if you are already fatigued or are recently recovering from an illness. In response to these conditions your immune system is compromised, which makes you far more likely to experience a severe allergic response to allergens.

126.   Be sure to clean every surface in your home on a regular basis. If you are the one suffering from allergies, be sure to wear a mask while cleaning. Since you will be stirring the allergens up as you clean, the mask will help keep you from breathing them in.

127.   Take caution when reading the newspaper. This may sound crazy, but if you often have allergies that irritate your skin, your newspaper might be hurting you. Try sticking your newspaper in the oven for a few minutes to bake the ink on the paper more, and you will experience less skin allergies on your fingers and hands.

128.   If you have carpeting anywhere in your home, be sure to take the time to vacuum it a few times a week. Also do not be stingy when you purchase a vacuum. Spend a little more to get a good quality vacuum and make sure that it has a HEPA (high efficiency particulate air) filter which will help trap allergens.

129.   Skip intense workouts during allergy season. When you are in an intense workout session, you

are likely to breathe more deeply, and more quickly. That means you are probably going to inhale much more pollen than usual. Which means you have a greater chance of experiencing allergy symptoms.

130.   Shower and change your clothes before going to bed every night. Be sure to thoroughly shampoo your hair. This will eliminate the buildup of allergens you acquire through the day. This also helps from spreading allergens, like dust and pollen, to your bed and making allergy symptoms worse overnight.

131.   Try your best to stay away from foods like dairy that can leave you congested. Although you may enjoy yourself very briefly with some rich dairy foods like ice cream. You can pay for it later when with a bad allergic reaction that can leave you congested for days.

132.   Be sure that you are drinking enough fluids (preferable water) when your allergies are flaring up. Fluids help flush out mucus from allergy symptoms while also keeping you hydrated. However, too much water can also flush out minerals your body needs, so be sure to take a multivitamin as well.

133.   If you are someone who is sensitive to getting a lot of allergies, then make sure you always carry some type of cloth or tissue. Do not be that person with a runny nose that does nothing about it. Be prepared at all times.

134.   To reduce your day to day allergies consider investing in an air purifier for your bedroom. While you are sleeping, you can have the air purifier create an allergen-free environment that will actually help clear your lungs, preparing you for the next day when you may come into contact with allergens elsewhere.

135.   Use hypo-allergenic cases for your pillows to keep dust mites from aggravating your allergies while you sleep. These cases seal the mites out of your pillow, yet remove easily for washing. Dust mites are a major cause of indoor allergies, so this simple step can save you a lot of suffering.

136.   Did you know that those whimsically named "dust bunnies" are really just jumbles of horrifying substances, including pet hair and dander, dust mites, and their feces and even insect parts? They are allergy attacks waiting to happen! Get rid of them on a daily basis, using a broom or vacuum.

137.   When you constantly battle allergies, it pays to devote a little extra time to cleaning the areas in which you live, work and play. For example, you should regularly wipe down any surface that you touch frequently like keyboards, countertops, door knobs and appliances. This reduces the amount of allergens that you come into contact with daily.

138.   When it comes to allergies, are you aware that even your own body can be making problems worse? It could be true! Over the course of the day, your hair, skin and clothing may become covered in pollen, mold, dust and other allergens. When you are finished with your day and climb into bed, these allergens can make breathing complex. A solution is to shower prior to bed and put on clean clothes before retiring for the night!

139.   For many allergy sufferers, it is impossible to effectively treat symptoms on their own. When the effects of seasonal and other allergies become too much to bear, it is wise to seek the assistance of a medical professional. By consulting with a specialist, you will have greater access to useful diagnostic tools and prescription treatments that would, otherwise, be unavailable to you.

140.   Wash your pillowcases on a regular basis, if you suffer from allergies. Pillowcases tend to collect dust, pollen, and other allergens that could really affect you. Washing them and your other linens can prevent this from happening. If you can, try to purchase non-allergenic pillows cases, sheets and other bedding.

141.   Some people assume that using a humidifier is good for allergy sufferers. If you have a carpet or rug in your room, mold spores can grow there thanks to the humidifier. Nasal saline spray administered at bedtime is a far better idea.

142.   If you are severely allergic to a certain kind of seafood, you may experience a reaction without even ingesting it. Steam that arises from seafood that is being prepared or boiled may be enough to trigger a serious allergic reaction. Never cook with an ingredient that you are allergic to, even if you do not intend to eat it.

143.   When it is the height of allergy season, it's a good idea to wear your hair naturally and not use excessive hair products. Whenever you are outside, allergens can get trapped and stuck in your hair. Hair products can cause cause your hair to collect allergens.

144.	Your doctor may hold the key to helping you treat your allergy symptoms. Some over-the-counter medications and nasal sprays may not be strong enough to actually help your symptoms. Your doctor may feel that it is best that he or she write you a stronger prescription. Just make sure you tell your doctor about any health conditions you have.

145.	Make sure that your home is free of irritants as much as possible when coping with allergies. You should vacuum frequently with a vacuum that is equipped with a HEPA (High-Efficient Particulate Air) filter. This will help capture airborne particles, such as mold, dust, pollen, bacteria and dust mites, which are common causes of allergies.

146.	Kitchens are breeding grounds for mold, which can torment would-be chefs who have mold allergies. To discourage the growth and spread of this unwanted intruder, always use an exhaust fan while preparing food on the stove or in the oven. This draws excess moisture from the air, which makes it difficult for mold to grow.

147.	It may be tempting to move elsewhere to try to avoid the allergens that are causing your allergies. When this thought crosses your mind, remember that the most common allergy causing plants (grass and ragweed) are found everywhere. So a move to a different climate may not help your situation.

148.   Time your outings. Statistics have shown that pollen count is affected by time of day, temperature, rain, and humidity. The worst times to be outdoors are between 10 in the morning and 4 in the afternoon, especially on days that are windy, hot and dry. So if you really want to spend some time outdoors, wait until the late afternoon.

149.   Find an allergen forecast and use it to plan your day. The Weather Channel and some other major outlets provide information about pollen activity and other information about allergens. These forecasts can not only let you know which days are likely to be worst for your symptoms, but they can pinpoint the worst times of day to be outside.

150.   One way to keep allergies under control is, to make sure that all of the surfaces in your house are cleaned. This is good to do because you will limit the amount of exposure you will have to dust, and other particles that may cause allergy

outbreaks. Limit the amount of chemicals that you use by just cleaning with a damp rag.

151.   Change your bedding frequently, and wash using hot water. Pollen, dust, and other allergens can stick to your clothing and hair and can get deposited on your bedding. Sheets and pillowcases may appear clean, but can harbor irritants that will affect you while you sleep. These allergens easily wash away when the items are cleaned in hot water.

152.   If you suffer from allergies, it is best that you do not have carpets in your home. And if you do insist on having carpets, get allergy care ones. Carpets hold dusts and other particles that will send your allergies out of control, even if you do clean them often.

153.   People can be affected by allergies at any age. Many Baby Boomers grew up without access to allergy tests, and other medical resources. They have lived with allergic symptoms for decades. Allergic reactions often manifest differently in seniors than in young people. For example, older adults may experience itching, and mild swelling, but not localized redness. As a result, many assume that the cause of discomfort is something other than allergies. An allergy test can help

seniors to identify allergens, and live their golden years to the fullest.

154.   For those who love the idea of toiling in their own vegetable garden, allergies caused by mold and pollen can seem especially oppressive. Fortunately, this does not mean would-be gardeners have to give up their hobby altogether. Instead, they must outwit outdoor allergens. The ideal time to garden is immediately after a storm when rainwater flushes away clouds of pollen, spores and other allergens. Alternately, one could use a garden hose to spray the area in which they plan to work.

155.   If your allergies are accompanied by a harsh, hacking cough, irritation in the throat is probably to blame. This is especially common in those who fight post-nasal drip or mouth breathing. In many cases, the problem becomes more pronounced during the night. When this happens, try using pillows to prop you up in a half-reclining position while you sleep. If you can sleep while sitting upright, that's even better.

156.   Too many people let their allergies limit what they can do. This doesn't have to be the case. There is no reason to stop taking those hikes you used to love or stop playing games with your

kids out in the yard. Fight those allergies and get a good handle on them. Make an appointment with an allergist and figure out the best treatment that will help you the most.

157.   Colorants are often allergens, so avoid any product containing them. This comes down to even your toilet paper that may have designs dyed into them. Use white paper products only, like paper towels, to see if that relieves allergy symptoms.

158.   Olive trees have become popular in many western states. Unfortunately, the trees also produce a lot of pollen. Therefore it is important to identify these trees and protect yourself. A lot of people find that using water hoses on trees with a lot of pollen can help tame the pollen.

159.   Allergy symptoms may be making your little one miserable and irritable, but that doesn't mean he's necessarily ready to take liquid medications without a fight. If your child complains about the taste, ask a pediatrician or pharmacist if you can mix the medication with fruit juice to mask the taste.

160.   People who suffer from food allergies are generally the ones who need to be the most

careful. While other types of allergies can be annoying, food allergies tend to be the most fatal. This is especially true of people who suffer from allergies to shellfish or nuts, such as shrimp or hazelnut.

161.   A good way to reduce your exposure to allergens is to close your windows and doors in the morning and night. Many of the common allergens are at their peak during these times of the day. Most outdoor allergens are pollen. Natural sources like pollen are at their highest levels at these times of the day.

162.   Kitchens are breeding grounds for mold, which can torment would-be chefs who have mold allergies. To discourage the growth and spread of this unwanted intruder, always use an exhaust fan while preparing food on the stove or in the oven. This draws excess moisture from the air, which makes it difficult for mold to grow.

163.   Find out what is causing your allergy symptoms. Many people focus on the itching and sneezing, but it's important to get to the root of the problem. Take a look at your environment and discover what is triggering your allergies. You might be allergic to more than one thing, so take care and investigate all possible causes.

164.   When ever you are cleaning your house, use a dust mask. This will help keep away the dust, pollen, and dust mites that are scattered in the air, as you clean out of your system. Most supermarkets have these in the cleaning supplies aisle. If they don't, home improvement stores sell them in bulk.

165.   Get tested by a doctor to find out what exactly you are allergic to. You can try to find out on your own, but seeing a doctor and having the appropriate blood tests are the only ways to know for sure. Once you have pinpointed the cause of your allergies, you can better treat them.

166.   If you suffer from allergies, it is best that you do not have carpets in your home. And if you do insist on having carpets, get allergy care ones. Carpets hold dusts and other particles that will send your allergies out of control, even if you do clean them often.

167.   Mold is one of the most common allergens, and the bathroom is the room most prone to growing it. This is due to the moisture from showers and bathtubs. To keep mold to a minimum, always turn on the bathroom fan. Try

painting with a mold-resistant paint that, can be found anywhere that sells paint.

168.   When you constantly battle allergies, it pays to devote a little extra time to cleaning the areas in which you live, work and play. For example, you should regularly wipe down any surface that you touch frequently like keyboards, countertops, door knobs and appliances. This reduces the amount of allergens that you come into contact with daily.

169.   There are a lot of antihistamines and allergy products on the market you can get without a prescription. If purchasing a new product for the first time, look for the smaller travel sizes so you can test it out or request complimentary office samples from your doctor. If the product doesn't help you reduce your symptoms, then you can try another without wasting too much money.

170.   If allergy season has made your eyes dry, itchy and irritated, a cold compress may be just the thing you need to find relief. Applying a chilled gel pack, eye pillow or cloth over your eyes can reduce swelling within minutes. This also works wonders for eliminating unsightly redness; it is in addition extremely relaxing!

171.   If you have allergies and own pets, it may be difficult to determine whether or not they are the cause of your problems. In order to find out, have a doctor test you for an allergy to pet dander. If you are allergic to your pets, you can usually make a few changes rather than give them up.

172.   If you've exhausted your options and your allergy symptoms aren't letting up, it's best to seek out advice from a physician. They can help you find medication that can manage and control your symptoms. They may also be able to suggest additional ways you can cope with your allergies.

173.   If you are severely allergic to a certain kind of seafood, you may experience a reaction without even ingesting it. Steam that arises from seafood that is being prepared or boiled may be enough to trigger a serious allergic reaction. Never cook with an ingredient that you are allergic to, even if you do not intend to eat it.

174.   Invest in an air purifier. An air purifier, especially in the bedroom, can help make a person with allergies much more comfortable. These units circulate air similar to a fan, while filtering out dust and other air pollutants. For the

best results, look for a unit that features a HEPA filter.

175.   Consider removing carpeting from your home, and going with wood or laminate flooring. Carpet allows dust mites to build up, and this can irritate allergies. If possible, remove the carpeting from your home, and replace it with laminate or wood flooring. Thiss prevents extra build of of allergens in your home.

176.   Clean your home from top to bottom at least once per year, preferably in the spring. A deep cleaning can eliminate dust, dander, mold and other allergens. If this type of cleaning is too daunting, hire a service to complete the job for you. You can maintain the results yourself or schedule regular visits from the cleaning service, after the initial deep-clean.

177.   Make a saltwater nasal spray at home if you suffer from allergies. This can greatly help any nasal congestion you have. To do this, simply mix a half a teaspoon of salt with 8 ounces of water into a squirt bottle. Then, just use the spray in your nose like you would have with any other nasal spray.

178.   When you want to go on a vacation, don't just randomly pick a place to go. This can be a great risk if you have an allergy sufferer in your family. Before deciding on a destination, research pollen counts, weather conditions and other things that could trigger allergies.

179.   Get tested by a doctor to find out what exactly you are allergic to. You can try to find out on your own, but seeing a doctor and having the appropriate blood tests are the only ways to know for sure. Once you have pinpointed the cause of your allergies, you can better treat them.

180.   Try your best to stay away from foods like dairy that can leave you congested. Although you may enjoy yourself very briefly with some rich dairy foods like ice cream. You can pay for it later when with a bad allergic reaction that can leave you congested for days.

181.   You can reduce the amount of exposure you have in your home to potential allergens. You should keep your windows, and doors closed to prevent pollen from entering your home. You can take a quick shower after returning from outdoors to remove pollen from your eyelashes, hair and skin. You should also change clothing

and put the clothes that you wore outdoors in closed hamper.

182.   If you suffer from allergies, change your pillowcase regularly, at least once a week. A pillowcase harbors dander and dust, which can trigger allergy symptoms. Since your face is directly in contact with a pillowcase for several hours a day, having one that triggers your symptoms will make you feel miserable. Wash your pillowcases in hot water, and change them out regularly.

183.   If you are troubled by different allergies in your home, try putting a dehumidifier or two in the common areas of your living space. Reducing the humidity by at least half can really cut down on potential mold growth, and mold is known to be a big contributor to allergies.

184.   Before you commit to allergy injections, understand that having these shots will not eliminate the allergy itself. Actually, these injections increase your body's threshold. As a result, you can tolerate greater exposure to the allergen before you start to experience discomfort or an allergic reaction. A realistic idea of the results can help you to make the decision whether or not the procedure is worth it.

185.   Make your home a little more allergy-free by implementing a no-shoes policy. Why? Because shoes come in from outdoors and carry with them dirt and pollen among other things, only adding to the indoor allergens you are already trying to eliminate. When guests come, offer them slippers or socks you keep especially for this purpose!

186.   Wash your pillowcases on a regular basis, if you suffer from allergies. Pillowcases tend to collect dust, pollen, and other allergens that could really affect you. Washing them and your other linens can prevent this from happening. If you can, try to purchase non-allergenic pillows cases, sheets and other bedding.

187.   Keep an eye on your stress levels. Believe it or not, something as simple as stress can have a very negative impact and actually cause allergies to get worse. It is is truth, even more so for those who have asthma. A rise in stress can increase the likelihood of an asthma attack or allergy outbreak. Although, it won't cure allergies, it will help the amount of allergic reactions experienced.

188.   When looking at your local weather forecast, if you see that pollen is going to be high, take your allergy medication in advance. Why wait until pollen gets too bad to take your medication? Instead, take it in advance, so that you do not have to suffer when going outdoors for the day.

189.   Try using a dehumidifier in your home and keeping your humidity in your home below 45 percent. This setting will inhibit any mold growth in your home and keep it an allergy safe environment for you and your family. You can buy a humidity meter at any hard ware store.

190.   Many children have difficulty swallowing medication in pill or capsule form, making it a major undertaking to get allergy medication down without tears or a fight. If this sounds like your little one, consider switching to an orally disintegrating tablet. These lozenges dissolve quickly on the tongue and taste like fruit or mint.

191.   Kitchens are breeding grounds for mold, which can torment would-be chefs who have mold allergies. To discourage the growth and spread of this unwanted intruder, always use an exhaust fan while preparing food on the stove or

in the oven. This draws excess moisture from the air, which makes it difficult for mold to grow.

192.   Few things are more irritating to the eyes and nose than exposure to cigarette smoke (first- or second-hand). However, many people mistake this irritation caused by smoke for an allergen and take allergy medications to counter the effects. Because smoke is not a true allergen, these treatments will not have any effect on the symptoms.

193.   Take the time to clean your home thoroughly. It is common for individuals to be vulnerable to multiple types of allergens, and therefore thoroughly cleaning your home is a great way to manage all symptoms. Endeavor to clean your surroundings with great frequency.

194.   Consider taking an over the counter medicine to battle allergy problems. Medicine may clear up any allergy problems you have. Before choosing which medicine is right for you, consult your doctor to make sure it won't affect any medication you are currently taking. Your doctor may also recommend an allergy medicine to you.

195.   While you may be tempted to bundle up with a wool blanket during the cold winter months, think twice if you suffer from allergies year-round. Compared with other materials, wool collects and locks in immense amounts of dust, as do down comforters. Instead, opt for bedding that is made only of synthetic materials.

196.   Allergies can wreak havoc on your eyes, which may cause you to rub or tug at the skin around your eyes. Any allergens, bacteria or problematic substances will be transferred from your fingers to your eyes, which may increase your discomfort. Always remember to wash your hands thoroughly after handling pets, plants or other common sources of allergens.

197.   To reduce your day to day allergies consider investing in an air purifier for your bedroom. While you are sleeping, you can have the air purifier create an allergen-free environment that will actually help clear your lungs, preparing you for the next day when you may come into contact with allergens elsewhere.

198.   For people who suffer from seasonal allergies, the best way to reduce your symptoms is to leave the outdoors outside. When you are in your car, drive with the windows up. At home,

close windows and use the air conditioner. If you do go outdoors, then you should change your clothes when you come home because it will collect allergens.

199.   Allergy sufferers can benefit by using a neti pot. A neti pot is used to rinse nasal passages and by doing so, it can help with allergy symptoms. Fill the pot with lukewarm, distilled water and a teaspoon of table salt to create a saline solution. Lean your head to the side, and pour the water into one nostril at a time. This is a great and natural method for allergy relief.

200.   Shower before bed, taking special care to wash your hair thoroughly. Pollen, dust, and other allergens can get trapped on your skin and in your hair as you go through your day. If you normally shower in the morning, consider switching to an evening schedule. This will give you the chance to remove these irritants before bed, allowing you to have a restful night's sleep.

201.   If you have allergies, it is important that you keep the humidity in your home to a minimum. You can do this by setting up a dehumidifier in whichever rooms you are frequently in. One of the worse things for an allergy sufferer is

humidity, so stay away from it as much as you can.

202.   Make your home a little more allergy-free by implementing a no-shoes policy. Why? Because shoes come in from outdoors and carry with them dirt and pollen among other things, only adding to the indoor allergens you are already trying to eliminate. When guests come, offer them slippers or socks you keep especially for this purpose!

203.   If you have allergies and are facing yard work, protect yourself with a mask! Any inexpensive painter's mask will help to keep pollen from the grass and flowers from bothering you. Wear one whenever you have to kick up leaves, mow the lawn or trim hedges, and you should reduce the symptoms you experience.

204.   When you know allergy season is going to begin, use this time to take a vacation. Obviously, spending time outside is going to make your allergies act up, and you do not want to have to sit inside all of the time. Go to a beach location, where you can be allergy-free.

205.   Going for a run around the neighborhood may make you feel wonderful and alive, but

pollen and spores in the air can quickly spoil the experience. This is especially true if you are already fatigued or are recently recovering from an illness. In response to these conditions your immune system is compromised, which makes you far more likely to experience a severe allergic response to allergens.

206.   Do not allow your seasonal allergies keep you from the joys and health benefits of a good run outdoors. The best time to engage in physical activities outdoors is immediately after a rainshower. Rain tames clouds of pollens, spores and mold and makes you less likely to encounter high allergen levels.

207.   While driving to school or work during a peak allergy season, set your vehicle's air-conditioning unit to "recirculate." This setting cleans and cools the air without drawing in pollen or spores from outside. Whenever you take your car in for an oil change, ask the mechanic to replace your air filter as well.

208.   Set a limit on how many carpets and rugs are allowed in your home. No matter how much you try to clean them, they can harbor allergens. If you want rugs to add some softness to a room, be sure you can wash them to remove allergens.

209.   Invest in hypoallergenic mattress pads and pillowcases. Regardless of how often you wash your sheets, without any protection, your pillows and mattresses are going to gather dust and other allergens. Hypoallergenic mattress pads and pillowcases act as an impenetrable barrier - keeping your bed a safe haven from your allergies.

210.   Always be sure that you are receiving the proper medications for your children if they suffer from severe allergies of any type. A note from a pediatrician explaining the allergies your child has can be useful. The school nurse should keep the medication on hand for regular dosing and in case of emergencies. Be sure to provide the school with a list of your child's allergens, and keep an additional copy in his or her backpack.

211.   If you can spare the added expense, hire another person or a professional lawn care service to take care of all of your landscaping needs. The acts of mowing, raking and weeding can stir up an immense amount of mold, pollen and dust, making you more vulnerable to an allergy attack.

212.   When your allergies are acting up, do not drink or eat any dairy products. These foods and drinks increase the amount of phlegm you have, which is just going to make you feel worse. Foods and drinks you want to avoid are milk, yogurt, and cheese. There are many non-dairy versions of your favorite dairy products.

213.   One way to keep allergies under control is to keep the air inside your house clean. This can be accomplished by changing your heater. and air conditioner filters. You can run an air cleaner inside your house. Cleaning your air filters this will not only improve the air inside your home, but ensure that your central air blowers run properly.

214.   Smog can make many people have allergies in bigger cities. If you live in the city and always find yourself congested then consider taking a trip outside of the city for a week. See how you feel, and when you return you may realize all of the smog is giving you allergies.

215.   Keeping your home free from crumbs, especially in hidden areas such as behind or underneath kitchen appliances, is a great way to reduce allergy symptoms. This is crucial because with crumbs comes pests, such as cockroaches

and mice. Not only do mice come with dander, but droppings can cause additional allergic reactions.

216.   If you suffer from allergies in the spring as trees, and flowers begin to bloom, try to minimize the amount of pollen in your home. Wash your sheets, and pillowcases every week with hot water. Vacuum your rugs, or carpeting twice a week. Wash your hair at night to get rid of any pollen that has accumulated

217.   Use a once-a-day allergy medicine to relieve your allergy symptoms before you experience them. You can take one pill in the morning. and you will not feel the effects of your allergies all day long. There are several different brands available, mostly over-the-counter, so find one that works for you.

218.   If you suffer from allergies, it is best that you do not have carpets in your home. And if you do insist on having carpets, get allergy care ones. Carpets hold dusts and other particles that will send your allergies out of control, even if you do clean them often.

219.   Avoid line-drying your clothing, or linens if you suffer from allergies, especially during the

spring. While the smell and feel of fresh, line-dried laundry can be a treat. It can also make you miserable when you bring in pollen from outdoors. Use the clothes dryer when pollen levels are at their peak.

220.   Before you commit to allergy injections, understand that having these shots will not eliminate the allergy itself. Actually, these injections increase your body's threshold. As a result, you can tolerate greater exposure to the allergen before you start to experience discomfort or an allergic reaction. A realistic idea of the results can help you to make the decision whether or not the procedure is worth it.

221.   Consider going without carpet. Putting in hardwood floors instead of having carpet will ensure that no allergens are lurking just under your feet. If your carpeting is wall-to-wall, replace it with wood, tile or laminate floors if you can afford it. Doing so will greatly reduce a concentration of allergy triggers in your home. If getting rid of your carpet isn't feasible, vacuum daily instead.

222.   Consult with your doctor if all of your OTC and home remedy efforts have failed. A doctor can prescribe a stronger medication to bring

relief from your symptoms. A healthcare professional will also be able to offer additional insight into lifestyle changes or practices that can improve your chances for success.

223.   People who suffer from food allergies are generally the ones who need to be the most careful. While other types of allergies can be annoying, food allergies tend to be the most fatal. This is especially true of people who suffer from allergies to shellfish or nuts, such as shrimp or hazelnut.

224.   Many doctors are more than willing to write prescriptions for the latest and greatest allergy medications, but some are utterly clueless about the high price tag. If you are having a hard time paying for these medications, ask for samples or contact the drug manufacturer to inquire about patient assistance programs.

225.   If your child is allergic to peanuts, it is vital to keep his or her school informed of this. Talk to the principal and all teachers to make sure they are aware of the allergy. Also, have them keep a note on file to cover all the bases. Many foods contain "hidden" peanut oils or peanut products. Even some cookies and crackers

contain peanut product, so be diligent, for your child's sake.

226.   Pay attention to the pollen count reports. Since pollen counts report how many grains of pollen were counted in a specific area, over a specific time frame, they could be used to determine how much pollen is floating around in the air on the given day. This could be used to determine how much time you might want to spend outside.

227.   If you have allergies, one hidden danger to you may be the damp areas of your home. Places like basements and garages will harbor mold and instigate attacks, so either avoid these areas during the damp season, or see that they are thoroughly cleaned with a simple solution of bleach and water.

228.   Consider taking an over the counter medicine to battle allergy problems. Medicine may clear up any allergy problems you have. Before choosing which medicine is right for you, consult your doctor to make sure it won't affect any medication you are currently taking. Your doctor may also recommend an allergy medicine to you.

229.   Check on the pollen count every morning. When you know exactly what the pollen count is you can organize your day. If things look particularly high in the morning, try to avoid something like jogging or running errands. The pollen count will decrease later in the day, so put things off until then if possible.

230.   For some, even a miniscule amount of pollen is able to spark allergic episodes, and therefore making any reductions at all can be beneficial. When you go into your home, take off your shoes and your coat so you do not bring pollen into your home. Another way to reduce the amount of pollen that makes it into your house is to wash your hair immediately after returning home.

231.   If you have an allergy to pollen, keep an eye on weather reports to find out when the pollen count is high. During these times, stay indoors as much as possible with windows and doors closed. You may get a little "cabin fever," but you may feel healthier by not being over-exposed to allergy-irritating pollen.

232.   If you have been outside during the day and you suffer from allergies, be sure you are taking a shower right before you go to bed. This helps to

wash off all the pollen and other allergens from your body and hair, so it doesn't cause you issues when you are trying to sleep.

233.   To reduce allergies, lower the exposure your eyes get to bright light, particularly sunlight, by wearing items such as sunglasses and hats. Many times, allergic reactions are aggravated when your eyes are exposed to an intense spectrum of light. Preventing this exposure is key to lowering the possibility of an unfavorable response to allergens that may be present.

234.   Use hypo-allergenic cases for your pillows to keep dust mites from aggravating your allergies while you sleep. These cases seal the mites out of your pillow, yet remove easily for washing. Dust mites are a major cause of indoor allergies, so this simple step can save you a lot of suffering.

235.   People who suffer from allergies often have dry, irritated nasal passages that are prone to redness, itchiness and bloody noses. To keep these airway's moist, use a spray of saline solution in each nostril several times per day, then apply a thin layer of petroleum jelly inside the nostrils to keep moisture in.

236.   Mold is one of the most common allergens, and the bathroom is the room most prone to growing it. This is due to the moisture from showers and bathtubs. To keep mold to a minimum, always turn on the bathroom fan. Try painting with a mold-resistant paint that, can be found anywhere that sells paint.

237.   Think about taking the carpet out of your house. Pollen and dust tends to gather on carpets. If your carpeting is wall-to-wall, replace it with wood, tile or laminate floors if you can afford it. There will be a substantial difference in how much allergens you breathe in. If you cannot switch to these kinds of floors, vacuum everyday.

238.   Athletic types who struggle with allergies, often find themselves dreading their daily jog around the neighborhood when pollen counts are high. While some level of pollen will always be in the air at any given time, there is still hope. Pollen content is often at its highest between 5 a.m. and 10 a.m. Choose another period outside of this window, and you should have less trouble.

239.   When you know allergy season is going to begin, use this time to take a vacation.

Obviously, spending time outside is going to make your allergies act up, and you do not want to have to sit inside all of the time. Go to a beach location, where you can be allergy-free.

240.   If you are allergic to pet dander, designate at least one area in the house as a "pet-free" zone. Your bedroom is the most obvious choice. Keeping this area clean, and free from intrusions by your furry friends can significantly alleviate your allergy symptoms. The alternative, of course, is to designate a single area in which your pet can stay.

241.   In the first few months of their lives, household pets like dogs and cats generally have little to no dander. As they get older, shedding and dander problems become more pronounced. Because the animal has lived in the house up to that point, owners may be reluctant to believe their beloved pet is the cause of the sudden onset of allergic symptoms. An allergy test can help to identify the true culprit.

242.   Try limiting the amount of throw rugs and carpets that you have in your home. They attract large quantities of pollen and dust. Rugs add softness to your home decor, but make certain

they are washed often to prevent accumulation of allergens.

243.   Many people do not realize they might be exposing themselves to increased allergens just, by the way, they dry their clothes. If you suffer from allergic reactions to pollen, then hanging your clothes outdoors to dry can cause allergic reactions. When the clothes hang, they collect all the pollen that is blown in the breeze while drying.

244.   To avoid allergens in your bedding, a good tip is to use pillows made of synthetic materials rather than feather or cotton pillows. Dust mites will visit these pillows less than those with natural materials. It is important to get allergy covers for the pillows, and launder both the covers and pillows often.

245.   Keep your windows closed when pollen counts run high. It is important to get fresher air circulating through your home, but do it when pollen counts are lowest. Usually this is between 10 am and 3 pm. Air your home out before or after these hours.

246.   If you are one of the millions who suffer from allergies, you probably should change your

air filters in your air conditioner every month. The manufacturers usually will say to change every three months, but if you have problem allergies, you should do it more often to ensure all allergens are trapped before being dispersed through your home.

247.   If you suffer from allergies, you need to carefully choose which laundry detergents you use. Certain brands of detergents can trigger allergy symptoms. If you find that all detergents bother your allergies, you could always wash your clothing, and your linens with baking soda. Also, allow your clothing to air dry rather than using a dryer.

248.   If you suffer from annoying allergies, don't use a clothes line to dry your laundry. As nice as it is to have the natural scent of clothes dried outside by the wind and sun, you will also have an abundance of sneezes inducing pollens. So use an electric dryer whenever you can!

249.   During certain times of year, people who suffer from allergies have reactions to things in their environment. If you are having symptoms that you think are related to allergens in your environment, consult your physician to try to identify the culprit. Taking over the counter

remedies may work to some extent, but you are better off seeing a doctor to advise you on your condition.

250.   Watch your local weather forecast to see if pollen is high for that day. If it is, it's best that you minimize your time spent outdoors. If you do want to go outdoors, make sure it's not between the hours of 5 and 10 A.M. This is the time when pollen is high.

251.   Determine why you itch. Sometimes it can be difficult to know whether the itchy, raised welts on your skin are hives or just insect bites. If the bumps appear all over your body, they are probably hives. Insect bites, on the other hand, appear in clusters and on the arms on legs. Topical products are ideal for either ailment; oral anti-histamine is recommended to treat allergies, but is not necessary for insect bites.

252.   Because mold grows in warm, damp environments, it is very common in organic gardening materials. Compost heaps are a significant source of mold spores and other allergens, which is very frustrating for allergy sufferers who prefer eco-friendly gardening techniques. While composting, always wear a

face mask. This allows you to do your dirty work without having an allergy attack.

253.   If at all possible, never open your windows during hours in which pollen count is at its highest. Pollen is looking for a place to land. It blows around with the wind and can even fit through those ridiculously tiny holes in your window screen. From around 10 in the morning until 3 in the afternoon, pollen is at its peak. After this time has passed, open up your windows so that your home can air out.

254.   Take caution when reading the newspaper. This may sound crazy, but if you often have allergies that irritate your skin, your newspaper might be hurting you. Try sticking your newspaper in the oven for a few minutes to bake the ink on the paper more, and you will experience less skin allergies on your fingers and hands.

255.   Buy a dehumidifier for your basement. If you have a damp basement, this can be a breeding ground for mold. You can avoid mold build up, which triggers allergies, by putting a dehumidifier in your basement. You may want to buy a humidity gauge, to figure out the type of dehumidifier you need.

256.   When you want to go on vacation, you might want to pick a place and just go! This might not be a good idea if you or one of your family members has serious allergy problems. It's a good idea to research the weather, pollen conditions, and other allergy concerns that you'll encounter before you finalize your travel plans.

257.   Almost everyone knows another person who claims to be allergic to practically every substance in the universe and experiences a laundry list of symptoms in response. Actually, the effects of an allergic reaction are limited to any combination of only three symptoms. These include swelling (edema) of the mucosal membranes and skin, increased mucus secretion and smooth muscle spasms. Knowing the true signs of an allergic reaction can help you to determine whether or not medical assistance is needed.

258.   While an allergy test can be useful in helping you to identifying the culprit of your allergy symptoms, there are certain times in which taking this test is ill-advised. For example, you should never agree to an allergy test when you are experiencing severe asthma symptoms. It is also best to avoid testing while in recovery from surgery, or illness. During these periods, your

body may not respond to the tests, as it would in good health.

259. You may have dry or itchy eyes, and want to scratch; however, avoid contact with your hands. Instead, use an antihistamine eye drop to treat the symptoms. Continuing to rub your eyes can lead to irritated follicles along your lash line, which can then result in the formation of recurrent allergic styes.

260. Being sure to dust the entire home weekly will help keep your allergies under control. A lot of people ignore dusting around the house but it doesn't take that much time to do and is healthy for you and your family.

261. Did you know that those whimsically named "dust bunnies" are really just jumbles of horrifying substances, including pet hair and dander, dust mites, and their feces and even insect parts? They are allergy attacks waiting to happen! Get rid of them on a daily basis, using a broom or vacuum.

262. If you must work, drive or otherwise function all day, stay away from allergy medications that induce drowsiness. A number of less-drowsy formulas are available now, such

as loratadine. These medications provide a safer way to control your symptoms on the days that you cannot nap in the middle of the afternoon.

263.   Dry your clothes indoors. While hanging clothes outdoors to dry is good for the environment, it is not so good, if you suffer from allergies. Laundry that is hanging outside acts as an efficient pollen catcher, ensuring that the next time you wear those clean clothes, you will be reaching for the antihistamines.

264.   If you suffer from allergies, it is best that you do not have carpets in your home. And if you do insist on having carpets, get allergy care ones. Carpets hold dusts and other particles that will send your allergies out of control, even if you do clean them often.

265.   Exercise at the right time of day. If you like to exercise outdoors, yet you are an allergy sufferer, there are things that can be done so you can still enjoy the experience. It's better to exercise outdoors in the early morning or later in the evening as the pollen levels aren't as high at these times and less likely to cause issues with your allergies.

266.   Limit the amount of throw rugs you have around your home. They can gather dust, dirt, pollen, pet dander, and other allergens. If you do have throw rugs around the home, make sure they are washable. You can do this every week when you are cleaning your home.

267.   If your child frequently complains of symptoms like a stuffy nose, or frequent sneezing, allergies may be to blame. Over time, these problems can make it difficult for your child to perform well in class, or reach their full potential. In these cases, allergy therapy may produce a marked difference in the way your child feels, and behaves.

268.   Be sure to wash your hair immediately when you get inside, if you suffer from allergies and there was pollen outside. You do not want to allow the pollen to stay in your hair for too long, as this can trigger your allergy symptoms. It is best to wash your hair twice.

269.   When you know allergy season is going to begin, use this time to take a vacation. Obviously, spending time outside is going to make your allergies act up, and you do not want to have to sit inside all of the time. Go to a beach location, where you can be allergy-free.

270.   If you are severely allergic to a certain kind of seafood, you may experience a reaction without even ingesting it. Steam that arises from seafood that is being prepared or boiled may be enough to trigger a serious allergic reaction. Never cook with an ingredient that you are allergic to, even if you do not intend to eat it.

271.   If you are going outdoors when allergy season is in full force, wear sunglasses. Sunglasses prevent pollen, and other allergy triggers from getting in your eyes. About one hour before heading outdoors, put eye drops in your eyes. This will prevent your eyes from getting red when you are outdoors.

272.   Move your garbage outside of your house. Rodents, insects and other vermin are attracted to garbage. Droppings from rodents can worsen allergy symptoms. It may be necessary to set traps if you are unable to eliminate vermin from your home by this method. If traps do not get rid of them, you may need to consider a rodent poison.

273.   Be sure to clean every surface in your home on a regular basis. If you are the one suffering from allergies, be sure to wear a mask while

cleaning. Since you will be stirring the allergens up as you clean, the mask will help keep you from breathing them in.

274.   If you find yourself battling rhinitis or seasonal allergies to pollen and spores, you should always keep the windows in your home closed if possible. At the very least, close them between the hours of 5 and 10 in the morning; this is the time of day in which plants release higher concentrations of pollen.

275.   When pollen is high, do not open your windows. Although allowing fresh air into your home is desirable, try not to do so when the pollen count is elevated during the day. This is usually between 10am and 3pm. You can let in the breeze after this time.

276.   Don't forget to take allergies into consideration when planning a vacation out of town. This is risky if you have allergies or one of your family members do. It's a good idea to research the weather, pollen conditions, and other allergy concerns that you'll encounter before you finalize your travel plans.

277.   While certain foods can hurt your allergies, other foods may be helpful. For instance, when

eating your favorite meal, add horseradish, chili pepper, and hot mustard. All of these work by cleaning out pollen and any other particles that you may have in your nose. It will clear your nasal passages.

278.   Monitor pollen forecasts and plan accordingly. If you have access to the internet, many of the popular weather forecasting sites have a section dedicated to allergy forecasts including both air quality and pollen counts. On days when the count is going to be high, keep your windows closed and limit your time outdoors.

279.   Change your bedding frequently, and wash using hot water. Pollen, dust, and other allergens can stick to your clothing and hair and can get deposited on your bedding. Sheets and pillowcases may appear clean, but can harbor irritants that will affect you while you sleep. These allergens easily wash away when the items are cleaned in hot water.

280.   If you suffer from allergies, you need to carefully choose which laundry detergents you use. Certain brands of detergents can trigger allergy symptoms. If you find that all detergents bother your allergies, you could always wash your

clothing, and your linens with baking soda. Also, allow your clothing to air dry rather than using a dryer.

281.   Mold is one of the most common allergens, and the bathroom is the room most prone to growing it. This is due to the moisture from showers and bathtubs. To keep mold to a minimum, always turn on the bathroom fan. Try painting with a mold-resistant paint that, can be found anywhere that sells paint.

282.   Allergen that can't be avoided is dust mites. Dust mites make their nests in your bedding, and they eat your dead skin cells. Talk about a nightmare! To combat these nuisances, encase mattresses and pillows in special zippered mattress covers and pillow cases. Then, wash bedding in hot water weekly, as hot water kills dust mites.

283.   If you suffer from allergies, choose a vacuum cleaner with disposable bags. While these vacuums are less ideal environmentally, they tend to be better for allergy sufferers because they trap dust, dander, pollen and more inside, rather than exposing you to the irritants when you empty a canister into the trash.

284.   Know the outdoor plants you are allergic to and check the calendar! You should know this information, if you can plan outdoor activities. This way, you can plan them on what days you should be taking your allergy medicine or packing some with you for the day.

285.   Watch your local weather forecast to see if pollen is high for that day. If it is, it's best that you minimize your time spent outdoors. If you do want to go outdoors, make sure it's not between the hours of 5 and 10 A.M. This is the time when pollen is high.

286.   Shower, and wash your hair before going to bed every night. Believe it or not, pollen can collect in your hair and on your body. Causing allergies to worsen overnight. Be sure to wash your body, and hair thoroughly before going to bed. This can be prevention for this happening.

287.   When you are under assault from pollen and mold, few things are more intimidating than the idea of mowing your lawn. To reduce the number of spores, and allergens stirred up by your lawnmower. Use a water hose to slightly dampen grass beforehand. You may end up working harder to get the job done, but almost

anything is better than an attack of allergy symptoms.

288.   Pinpoint your allergy triggers in order to prevent your symptoms. Your doctor or allergist can perform blood or skin tests to determine which substances cause an allergic reaction. This step helps you minimize your exposure to the substances that cause the most discomfort for you. You may also be able to narrow down your treatments to target specific allergens.

289.   If you own a pet and you suffer from allergies, you might be wondering weather your pet in to blame for your symptoms. Instead of assuming that your pet is the cause, visit an allergist to get tested. This does not mean that you have to re-home your pet, all it means is that you might need to make changes in your lifestyle.

290.   If your allergies are quite bad and keeping your home allergen free is not working as well as you hoped. You might want to consider taking some allergy medications. Talk to your doctor to find out if there is a medication out there that may work well to help combat some of your symptoms.

291.   Find out what is causing your allergy symptoms. Many people focus on the itching and sneezing, but it's important to get to the root of the problem. Take a look at your environment and discover what is triggering your allergies. You might be allergic to more than one thing, so take care and investigate all possible causes.

292.   If you have eye allergies then stop rubbing your eyes. Instilling an antihistamine in eye drop form can offer relief from these symptoms. If you continuously rub your eyes, it could cause an allergic stye.

293.   Pollen is more active between the hours of 5 a.m. and 10 a.m., so you should try to avoid being outside at that time, if you do not have to be. While pollen will be present at all times of the day, these are the hours where it is more abundant.

294.   One way to keep allergies under control is to be proactive with pollen control. This will ensure that you are not exposed to pollen for a longer duration and concentration than you normally would. This can be avoided by making sure that your sheets are washed regularly and that you clean your clothes and take a shower before going to bed.

www.ingramcontent.com/pod-product-compliance
Lightning Source LLC
Chambersburg PA
CBHW060753260726
48660CB00002B/595